NO MORE EXCUSES!

VOLUME 2

Take The Next Step Towards Healthy Living

DEITRA DAVIS (AUTHOR)

Introduction

This book is a continuation of volume one in which I really hope you enjoyed and found to be helpful.

I wrote volume two because there are so many different reasons we give or convince ourselves of everyday, in order to avoid committing to a healthier lifestyle, until I just couldn't fit it all into one book.

Helping others to overcome small obstacles by simply changing the way we think along with prioritizing is something that I have come to love

I hope you enjoy Volume two and find it as inspiring as Volume one.

Table of Contents

Contents

Chapter 1

I'm Too Fat To Exercise

Believing that you can't when you probably can would not be the best way to start in pursuing anything that you may have originally set your sites on. It's no different when it comes to getting in shape.

You first have to believe in yourself and believe in your abilities even though you haven't quite tapped into them.

Gaining weight, especially extreme weight gain, does not happen overnight. The same is true for losing it. The second thing you need to do is get a grip on your negative thinking and stop doubting yourself which is solely based on *"being too fat."*

Losing weight takes time and will also take patience on your part. Remember, it won't happen overnight, but if you stay focused, **IT WILL HAPPEN.**

There are plenty of ways to help you get moving, even if at a slower pace, so that you can reach your goals. Below are a few tips to get you started:

Don't Be In Such A Hurry

Take your time and don't be in such a hurry to see progress. Start at your own pace. A pace where you are most comfortable. By doing it this way, you won't fall off so easily. You will eventually get use to your new found daily activities. Consider limiting the amount of time you spend exercising per day. Maybe twenty to thirty minutes of physical activity will be enough. Try not to overdo it starting fresh out of the gate. This may only cause you to give up.

Exercising is a learned skill that will require patience to master.

Instead of worrying about how quickly your body will change, focus on today.

Find Something That Works For You

If you're worried about using equipment due to your weight, don't fret. This is where household items such as furniture could come into play and prove to be of much use.

For example: chairs that are positioned just low enough for

you to sit, then stand up, and repeat, could replace a strenuous squat. Even the bed can come in handy. I for one, like to lay in bed instead of using the floor or even a bench for things such as leg raises and crunches.

Beside, being much easier on my back, it's very comfortable. I'm sure you can come up with some ideas if you give it a little thought. This doesn't mean you should give up on equipment altogether because there are several that I'm sure could fit your needs.

A treadmill is one that will allow you to adjust your speed to as slow as you may need it to go. Then as you progress, take it up a notch. Stationary bikes are another great alternative allowing you to pedal at your own pace.

The main thing we want is to get moving. It really doesn't matter how you start.

If you have to start off really slow, *So What?* Like I previously stated, learning to exercise is a process and it takes time, even for smaller people. Never give up. You'll get better at it

Workout With A Motivator

Get with someone who is a very important part of your life.

Someone who encourages you to do more than you normally would.

Find that someone who will be right by your side no matter what you decide to do, but who will also push you along in a positive way.

Chapter 2

You're Already Small

Even though being small (in a healthy way), does associate with better health, you should still have a form of exercise within your weekly schedule.

Just like one might be fit but still looked upon as being overweight, the same goes for smaller frames. *Yes, you can be thin and yet be unfit.*

Being fit doesn't mean being small, it means being of good health both inside and out.

If you can say this about yourself, then hey, you're good to go. On the other hand, if you can do no more physically as if you were overweight, then I'd say you have work to do.

Understand that if you are not eating healthy and including productive activities into your schedule, then it doesn't matter if you are thin and small, big and tall, or all of the in between. You are still subject to a higher risk of avoidable diseases just as someone would who is twice your size.

Sure, it may not take as long to get into physical shape being that you're already small. That alone gives you a plus and may put you ahead of the game once you begin to start an exercise regimen, but you do need to start.

Having the wrong mentality about this entire process could possibly end with an undesirable outcome.

Besides that, exercising makes life feel more worth living. Ever feel fatigued, but you're not sick? Perhaps just a feeling of laziness, not wanting to get up and do anything? That could be a sign in itself.

Whenever you begin to feel any of these (symptoms), simply get up and get moving. Believe it or not, you will begin to feel much better.

Exercising helps you stay focused, build stamina, self-esteem, boost your energy level, as well as promote weight loss, (which we've already established you may not necessarily need). There are too many benefits that comes from exercising to count.

So why not give it a shot?

Get up and get moving

Chapter 3

I'm Too Busy

I'm too busy is one of the most common excuses for not exercising. I must admit that I have used it a time or two myself, but I had to realize that getting healthy and committing to a workout plan is just as important (if not more), than anything else that I do.

With all the activities that can flood your life, it's really easy to put ourselves last and never think twice about it. That is until something happens to change, making us put our health into a new perspective.

Why wait to be told we need to start exercising

(possibly by a doctor), before we make a go of it? Why wait until we realize that we can no longer do almost anything that we use to do, due to not properly taking care of ourselves?

The time is now to make a choice and say, *"Today is the day that I will begin to change my life."*

If it's important enough to you, then you will make the time, busy or not.

Below are some tips I am going to share with you in order to show you just how easy it can be to add a little physical activity into your busy schedule.

Exercise While You're At Work

Now before you say I must be out of my mind or you begin

to think about how impossible this will be to accomplish, depending on the type of job you may have, or the facility itself in which you earn your paycheck, there just might be a way.

If you have your own office or work in a cubicle, consider taking a small pair of hand weights with you. They can be easily kept in a drawer or somewhere out of site. Simple arm curls while sitting can go a long way in building those biceps.

If you work at a facility that has more than one level, you could go up and down the stairs during break. Skipping every other stair on your way up to mimic a lunge all while working the entire lower body.

Maybe your workplace comes equipped with a gym. If it does, all the better. You will only need to keep a bag of changing cloths with you at all times, (preferably in your car, office, or desk).

Before you start your shift, hitting the gym first may be ideal. What about your lunch hour? That's a perfect time to get a quick workout in and be prepared to return to your duties without skipping a beat.

The parking lot is a great place to get a few laps in as well. When I worked in the corporate world, I did it all the time. All it requires is a pair of comfortable walking shoes in which you should keep handy at all times to be able to put them on whenever you are ready to hit the pavement.

Perhaps a co-worker will tag along with you.

Getting in some exercise while at work can be done. Simply come up with some ways to help you get started, or feel free to use some of these tips.

Wake Up Earlier

Try waking up earlier than you normally would in order to get in a twenty or thirty-minute workout. It really doesn't have to be long and drawn out. If you work during the day, getting it in beforehand could be a really good thing.

You will have more energy to get you going *and you'll be able to stay more focused.*

This is something that I do as well, so I'm speaking from my own experience. I normally will get my *pump on* about an hour before I prepare for work and it really helps me get through my day.

Maybe going to sleep the night before a bit earlier than you normally would and perhaps setting an alarm clock, will help you to rise and shine. We all get busy, that's life. If we can make time for other things we feel are important, this should be one of them.

Make Use Of Time At Home

Admit it, we all have a little extra time to commit to exercise. There's an empty slot somewhere in our daily schedule that could be filled with taking better care of ourselves, but instead we choose to fill it with other things.

For example:

A long time spent on the telephone chatting away, or maybe texting non-stop.

The television is one I personally know so well. I love Netflix. You could say I'm a ride or die for that channel.

Social networking is also an extremely popular one. If a person can spend hours on the internet doing nothing really of importance, surely they can find time for a good, healthy, life changing workout.

So instead of just sitting around, how about committing to doing something that could change your world forever. It will only take a few minutes out of your day and your body will thank you for it.

Chapter 4

I'm Embarrassed

There are those who feel that attempting to workout at a gym is just far too embarrassing. They've just started out, have decided that *"Today is the day I'm going to make a change in my life for the better."*

They purchase a membership, walk in, then **Boom!** It hits them, **"I Can't Do This!"**

Looking around at all the people who seem to know exactly what they're doing. All of those fit bodies straddling every machine you could possibly imagine throws you into an uncomfortable state. So you attempt to push on anyway, but before long you find yourself heading for the door.

Before we quit and decide to never look back, try to identify what may be making you feel so uncomfortable and embarrassed.

Self-Conscious

Are you self-conscious about being out of shape? If you are, there are ways to get past this. As everyone seems to be so toned and in tune with their bodies, always remember, they had to start somewhere too.

We All Have To Start Somewhere

People don't just go from being completely out of shape to having the ultimate figure and good health at the snap of a finger. Rest assured, there are many people there who were in the same shape as you are now when they started. Use that as a form of motivation to keep going.

Feeling out of place is perfectly normal for a beginner, so don't beat yourself up about it.

The key to it all is to keep pushing and focus on your objective for being there in the first place and not on everyone else.

Everyone's Younger Than Me

This is one of the more typical reasons contributing to someone's embarrassment. It seems that everyone is so much younger than you. Maybe you're in your forties, fifties, or older, and everyone (that you've set your eyes on), seem to be barely tipping the age of twenty-five.

Well, that may be so, but notice my previous statement above... *(that you've set your eyes on)*. Rest assure there are plenty of people in the gym who are either equal or at least somewhere around your age

Never judge a book by its cover.

Meaning, just *because* someone may appear to be younger doesn't mean they necessarily are. Ever met someone who you assumed were entirely younger than they actually are?

Good health, habits, and physical activity sometimes play a vital role in someone's appearance.

If in fact you truly are a member of a gym which is filled with younger people and you feel uncomfortable, there are different types of gym settings that cater to people of different categories.

Consider shopping around for a different environment which will help you to feel a little more at ease.

I Don't Have Gym Attire

When we go to the gym, we're there for one thing only, (or at least we should be), and that's to workout. Too many of us tend to put more value on the clothing than the actual task at hand.

What you wear is not important at all just as long as you are comfortable.

Don't worry about making a fashion statement like so many tend to do. Just focus on why you are there. The spandex and all the other trendy outfits, (including name brands), being worn by some is not necessary unless this of course is your own personal preference.

Now if you truly don't have clothing worthy of your sweat, (because you will probably be doing a lot of that), consider buying yourself something that you can feel good in.

Keep it lose and comfortable so you can keep it moving.

CHAPTER 5

My Body/Weight Never Changes

If you are overweight and have tried to shed the pounds,
but it seems like nothing you do is working, I would first
suggest consulting with your physician about this issue.
On the other hand, if there is nothing physically wrong
preventing you from losing the weight, then maybe we have
something else to blame.

First you need to figure out what is really the problem. If
you are completely honest with yourself, then maybe you
will figure it all out.

Understand that if you are not eating a healthy diet and

applying exercise to the fullest of your potential, you won't see much of a change, if any at all.

"If you don't do anything different, don't expect anything different."

Are you eating less than you burn? One pound is equivalent to thirty-five hundred calories. This means you will have to burn off at least that amount of calories in order to lose a pound.

Trust me, it sounds harder than it really is. The hardest part is being patient, waiting for those pounds to drop off, because we're so full of anticipation over what the outcome will be.

We want it now and we don't want to wait.

It first involves watching your intake amount and applying

a little more exercise than you are presently doing.

Choosing to go on a diet would be completely up to you. Although I personally hate them. From my own experience, (and mines alone), I've found that most of them, I fail at.

Secondly, once you've lost the weight you desire and decide it's time to ditch the diet, there's a pretty good chance you'll begin to see those unwanted pounds creeping up on you once again.

Try measuring your food into portion sizes to ensure you don't overeat.

Clear your kitchen of high calorie snacks along with everything else that you know is unhealthy for you and replace it with more nutritional foods.

Now I don't proclaim to be a nutritionist by any means.

I'm simply letting you know what has worked and will surely assist you as well.

Ramp up your exercise and stay committed to your journey. Your body will have to adjust to all the changes. After it does, you should be well on your way to a new you.

Don't focus so much on what you can't see in the beginning. Instead, focus on why you started and how much better you will feel when it's over.

Eating healthy, (along with exercise), will allow you to eventually see those unwanted pounds begin to fade away.

(Give Yourself Credit in Knowing You've Started)

Conclusion

That about wraps it up for Volume 2. I really hope that after reading this book, you are able to see more clearly just how easy it can be to get around small obstacles standing in the way of you and your fitness goals. I also hope it will have given you more possible ideas (along with the ones presented), to help you stay focused. Be sure to join me once again in Volume 3 as I bring to you more profound reasons we use to avoid physical mobility.

No more excuses! No more procrastinating!

ABOUT THE AUTHOR

Deitra Davis is a mother of 3 fabulous children which have all grown to become wonderful adults. She presently enjoys online fitness coaching along with providing motivation to those in need of her help. Ms. Davis presently resides in Webster Texas and loves inspiring others to succeed in their fitness goals. Knowing she's helping others to live a healthier life drives her passion.

Feel free to learn more about Deitra at:

http://www.defitcoach.com
http://www.facebook.com/defitcoach

ONE LAST THING

If you have enjoyed this book or found it useful in any way, I'd be very grateful if you'd post a short review on Amazon. This is my very first publication and I would greatly appreciate hearing from you. Your support will make a difference.

I'll be reading all reviews personally in order to get your feedback and make my next book even better.

To leave a review:

http://www.amazon.com/dp/B01AQ32346?ref_=pe_242772780_160035660

www.ingramcontent.com/pod-product-compliance
Lightning Source LLC
Chambersburg PA
CBHW081543280526
45788CB00010B/3338